SKIN COLLECTION

Isobel Knight

chipmunkapublishing
the mental health publisher
empowering people

Isobel Knight

Published by
Chipmunkapublishing
PO Box 6872
Brentwood
Essex CM13 1ZT
United Kingdom

http://www.chipmunkapublishing.com

Chipmunkapublishing gratefully acknowledge the support of Arts Council England.

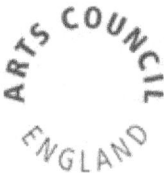

SKIN COLLECTION

Dedication

My love and thanks go to Nicola Hok who encouraged me with my writing after seeing some of my earlier poems, and for all her support throughout my ultimate recovery. I couldn't have done it without you!

My thanks go to Dr M. Hayward for her invaluable support during my Cognitive Analytical Therapy sessions (CAT) and for helping me to understand what I was doing, and how change could be possible.

Even though some of these poems might make upsetting reading, I hope that my mother and sister will understand that I love them both very much, and that this has been my way of processing some very difficult thoughts and emotions.

Finally my thanks go to Jason Pegler and Chipmunka Publishing for providing me with the opportunity to share my work, and to support those with mental health problems.

Isobel Knight

SKIN COLLECTION

Prelude:

People want to read my Poetry

People want to read my poetry.
Inside I am amused, inwardly laughing;
Are you sure you want to read my scrawl?
It makes Thomas Hardy read like a walk in the park

My poetry is not pretty; forget flowers and trees.
I am not going to make your day.
If you were feeling happy, you might want to get real.
I am going wipe the smile off your face.

You are going to a place that is deep and dark,
the very crevices of my soul.
Some of my words will make you weep,
Are you sure you want to proceed?

Isobel Knight

SKIN COLLECTION

At the Beginning

At the beginning we didn't know.
We were a clean slate and impressionable.
Nothing caused us pain, and it didn't occur to us to
mind.

Isobel Knight

Feelings

I wish I could tape them up and seal them in a box.
A lump of pure lead is closing up my throat, and an
ache is piercing my guts.

Happiness has slobbered out of my mouth and has
run far away.
I am feeling sickly and troubled, guilt groans inside
me.

I want to talk to someone, but I can't find the words.
Friends are empty voices and nobody understands
me.

Unhappiness seeps out of my pores and penetrates
my veins.
Trouble is a puzzling word.

Emotions are mysterious and overwhelming.
They are driving my life, crazy.

I try to encapsulate my feelings, but some things
can't be contained.

SKIN COLLECTION

Shades of Black

I can't stand this terrible flatness, of feeling sunken, empty and colourless.
I detest feeling indecisive
I loathe not wanting to do anything, my concentration like a butterfly.
I can't bear this feeling of horrific boredom, of only wanting to sleep.
I wish someone could let me die

I remember once wanting to do things, but not anymore.
For a long time now I just want to sleep – there is nothing to do.
To do anything is a superhuman effort

Isobel Knight

Thoughts of a Wet Day

It's relentless.
Needles of moisture dropping from slab-grey skies,
rhythmically smacking the ground timpanically.

There is an infinite supply;
The clouds are relieved of their tears,
It is a crying shame.

Water vibrates as it tumbles on the ground,
Gathering momentum collectively,
Puddles miserably form.

The air is subdued and day-time slowly mopes.
Splashes rebound and the spilling rain loudly
chatters.
I wait impatiently to go out.

SKIN COLLECTION

Don't Listen to Beethoven if you're Depressed

I tried to lift my spirits.
My moods were more up and down than a see-
saw.
The notes of a piano sonata were rattling past;
faster than speed.
My head was in a sand-pit.

In one ear and out of the other, the melody ran.
I tried to tame it and box it in, but it wouldn't listen.
It trickled past me and washed away;
My eyes glazed over and
My head rolled on the floor.

Music that I adore normally pacifies the beast in
me.
Beethoven usually touches my unfeeling heart.
Tuning into me, and matching my pathos.
Not today.
My head fell off, landing on deaf ears.

Isobel Knight

Stuck

It is all busy out there, and I am just stuck in a well
There is light out there somewhere
All I can see are bricks, infinitely and cosy.

God! Do you think if I shouted anyone would hear?
I can't stop crying.
The drip, drip of my tears are pooling around my feet;
There is not enough tissue to absorb their moisture.

I feel so excruciatingly sad, but I can't tell anybody about it.
No one understands, and I can't talk of it
I am just an act in a play that has gone on far too long
Change the scene.

The Crying Machine

Just like the reservoirs of windscreen wipers,
You keep your supply, enough to wipe out the rain.

When the button is pressed, emotions pour out.

Your body heaves.

Puddles collect in your cheeks and dribble in the descent of your nose.

Heavy sighs deplete deep within,
Ha Ha Ha, the crying machine.

Isobel Knight

Winter's Tale

In my head there is ebony black that is deeply compacted into every crevice of my being. It is smooth and solid and a liquid all at the same time, like the mercury in a thermometer. No oxygen can permeate, and the weight of the mercury-like substance is causing my neck to wilt like an over-burdened tree bough.

Because my head is so leaden down, very few thoughts are being processed, and everything is painfully slow. Very soon everything is going to grind to a complete halt.

The essence of me is being choked by the toxicity of this dark, congealed, tar-like mercury substance. Bit by bit I am being splintered; my memory is slow, my concentration is gone, I have less and less to say until the lights are dimming.... And eventually go out. Almost.

I am numb and no longer care about anything. Hunger signals that were once active lie dormant. My needs are obliterated and drowned out by the solid poison in my head. It silences my needs, my cares and my wants.

Like steam-rollers, my eyelids crash down upon the vacant blues of their irises. The relief to shut everything out is immense. I lie and wait for sleep to wave its veil of death and for me to succumb to slumber.

SKIN COLLECTION

Sleep blocks out all the noise and pain of my splitting head. It allows me for a few hours to remain in a death-like trance and not to be me. This is my most pleasurable time of day, because I do not know. Nothing happens, and I do not exist.

****

Upon the realisation of daylight, my eyes do not want to open. My body is still dead heavy with sleep, and a cannon-ball weight rolls across my stomach as I realise the emptiness I feel deep inside. The dense fog in my head shifts uncomfortably. I move gently, but my head is too painful, and the sensation of deep sleep persuades me to linger.

My horizontal desires and the pull of the unconscious allow me to remain under the spell of sleep. Any thoughts that I have are submerged under the dreams that I am having. The longer I stay under the duvet, the more vivid and exhausting the dreams become.

When I do get up, it is as if I am not yet of 'this world'. I am somewhere between the realms of inlets in my mind. Life is blurred around the edges. Somehow I am not 'real'. As I am coming to from this state, I often harm myself to rejoin the world.

The pain of the new scab being ripped off my skin jolts me back into the now. The blood flowing suggests that I really am alive. I now feel vaguely aware, and the blunt edge of nothingness is peeled away. I feel something. My skin is stinging, but I am also relieved and begin to wake up.

Sometimes, when I stare out of the window, or at the outside world, I feel extraordinary. I wonder how the world all came to be. I wonder how I came to be. I am very confused and feel sick as though I had been spun off a spinning top. What am I here for? What makes me move, and make decisions? How do I know where to go? What happened before I was here? What will happen when I go? I feel terrified, nauseous and overwhelmed. My mind is trying to understand something so vast, but makes me seem so inadequate and useless about everyday things.

Sometimes I think I am in a different world to everyone else. I am trying to understand other people's world, but it is not the same as the one that I am experiencing myself.

I want to be the same as everyone else. I want to be normal and do what I should be doing. Like a worn-out old computer, my brain is moving slower and slower. It is as if my brain needs a new memory, or a better hard-drive.

With the little capacity of functioning brain that I have left, I move slowly and laboriously through the day. I feel more and more detached from other people, the external world, and anything to do with it.

I only wish for death because nothing positive happens in my world. It remains a steely grey

SKIN COLLECTION

winter; barren and chilled. Winter, like an animal's tail, curls around me and encloses me like a circle and then it repeats its pattern. Again and again and again.

Isobel Knight

To Top it Off

Another fucking day.
A social occasion; time to hide.
Black, treacle galvanizes my skull
Go on, ruin it, I say.

With hands about my throat, I screw my top off.
There!
So easy.
The bastard rolls around the floor, casting aspersions.
I am so happy to be divorced.

Body and I go off to party, head wallows at home.
I wear a mask and have a wonderful time.
We were actually happy.
Together.
Body and mind.
I shovelled earth on top of my head.

SKIN COLLECTION

Oh for Dopamine

I am coming back now.
Grey matter takes over black hole.
White matter gives it a rinse, cleansing my soul.
Dopamine penetrates.

I grow, toweringly high.
Energy floods my being;
Electricity – I have the power.
The world is my oyster.

On the edge of insanity, I take the wrong jump
Craziness takes me too far,
It is unacceptable to be this high,
I am crushingly grounded
Off I go.....

Isobel Knight

Skin 1

Soft. Deeply soft.
Plump and podgy.
Spongy, yet wrinkled, with room for growth.
Fresh and brand-new.
Succulent, yet delicate.
Unblemished and unwritten.
Marshmallow bottomed,
Cherub-cheeked.

It will tell a story;
A chapter and verse.
You are young and impressionable.
I will leave my mark upon you,
So that I feel real.

SKIN COLLECTION

Skin 2

They say that it is scaly.
It is flaky and tiny bits fall off onto my clothing;
Repulsive, and itchy. Brillo-pad raw.
Upon pulling, particles of skin debris reveal a weeping soup;
Clear and dribbling, it falls down my arm.

The joints of my body are unfinished wood-work,
Sandpaper rough, creaky and aged.
I walk like a soldier.

Crepe bandages cover the damage,
Layers of cream lubricate this rotten tissue.

The snake in its armour shed.
I too wriggle free, discarding my old-self.

Isobel Knight

Skin 3

The dried blood is crusty and promisingly crunchy.
It hangs heavy on my skin,
My heart is daring me to open it.
Underneath it is a new secret, just waiting to be
exposed.

Adrenaline floods me as I try to prise the edges off
my prize.
Fluid glistens at the rim of my scab,
It cries tears as it knows what will happen next.

Slowly, my shell is peeled back. I am opening a
can.
The putrid flesh flashes a gooey orange and then
leaks red.
Anger explodes out of my skin, splashing against a
tide of limb.

Blood flows and then blots a piece of snow-white
tissue.
It bleeds violently.

I am relieved.
Although runny and moist, my skin is smooth.
The spot dries and becomes crispy and promisingly
crunchy.

SKIN COLLECTION

Skin 4

I am a walking freak show.
A dot-to-dot act, a giant clown.
Crazy excavations cover my skin,
Sealing numb emotions and a withered inner
person.

I wear a mask to get through the day,
Divorcing from the excruciating pain I am feeling;
Embarrassment, humiliation and shame.

What happened to your face?
Just a spot; an incredulous answer.

I shoulder their flinching stares and gapes of horror,
Their mirth, I am wearing, all over my fucking face.

Received slaps rebound my skin,
The hand reverberates, just as wind blows on the
old guitar string.
I am senseless and stupid; and very, very small.
I awake from the dream, but my nightmare
continues.

My face wears an insanity of broken skin.
Oozing wounds and disintegrating flesh are my lot.

Both of us go to school and face another day.

Isobel Knight

Skin 5

My fingers trace from one hole to another. Not caring to linger.
Each mark is a story in itself, a trial. A tribulation.
Pain.
Anguish
Torture
Scar me.
Their lasting mark an imprint on my face.

Misery, my fingers descend my neck, gliding with elegance and grace,
Slipping on to the mole-hills of my breasts, skiing down my chest.
Nipples resembling ball-bearings rolling along the ground.
I leave trails of nail marks encircling my thorax.

Suffering; my fingers skim emotionless along the contours of my body.
It feels as smooth as silk, with the coolness of a painted wall.
As my fingers glide south, they trace lands of long ago.
My navel squints above my muffin-top, only just able to see the fun.

I resent my southern triangle of darkness,
Curves and femininity.

Two pillars support my mass; Doric columns.
Sturdy, supple and strong, yet inelegant.

SKIN COLLECTION

Hairy and scaly, my lower-limb skin is sore and disfigured.
My anger has left its shadow on my shins,
Raw and broken skin disarrays.

My buttocks are dimpled, yet flat.
No cellulite, my hamstrings are firm and competent.
A flat landscape covers my back. It is smooth, yet characterless.
It lacks interest.

My skin *is* my story.
You will never get into my skin.
It does not fit my body.

Isobel Knight

Skin 6

The surface of the moon with its craters,
Round holes of terminal activity.
So it is with my skin; work completed.
Volcanic eruption.
Ended.

The aftermath remains; lumpy, damaged skin.
Knotted, flaying wood, ointment pink.
Experienced skin with a story;
Layers of epidermis with a tale to tell.

I am a disaster in recovery, with no aid pouring in.
Horribly exposed and vulnerable, I endeavour to
discover me,
My geography, lands and seas.

At rocket-point, I am re-launched.
I shed my space suit and apply my earth-face
I have some excavations to answer.

SKIN COLLECTION

Thoughts

My mind has burrowed deep underground. The soil is moist, dark and cold, and I am as flat as the East Anglian land. I am moving ever so slowly, like a worm crawling in the earth after a heavy meal. I am leaden in weight, and every move is a gigantic effort. To breathe is almost superhuman. My heart has dropped into my bowels, feeling like a knot in my middle. My head is full of black and death. Thought patterns are almost nil, and none of them are vocalising anything useful. The voices of my mind are suffocating me with negative information. I am drowning in my own despair.

The thoughts that I am having me are successfully convincing me that there is nothing worth being here for. Getting through the day is a massive effort. I am afraid at night that the blackness will overtake me and consume and destroy me. Thoughts of death pass me every time I wake at night. I try to block my ears to the scream of suicide taking tablets to give my poisonous head a rest.

In the morning I am totally exhausted as though I have been awake busy all week long. I am unable to make any decisions about anything and I flit like a butterfly between flowers around many activities, but never pause with one for long. I feel a gnawing discomfort in my stomach and feel that my throat is sealing up. I am not hungry at all. There is a lead pipe running through my digestive tract. I'll fill it with liquids and solids to fit in with others around me.

Isobel Knight

I am desperately hanging on to each moment at a time, fitting in with my surroundings, but I am finding it a terrible struggle. Everything has stopped still inside me. Time ticks by, but I am in a timeless void. I am suffocating in a tunnel and someone has put their hand over my face.

I absolutely cannot see where I am going now. For me there is no 'morrow because I am only stuck in today. Being fed, clothed and watered, living a nice house with a lovely partner and pussy cat should make me happy, so why do I feel so wretched?

Having some money in the bank and a book full of clients might help me to go on now if I had the energy. I feel that I need a holiday from myself. I need to leave this monster behind, to lock it away before it totally consumes me.

I am scared because I believe that I have accomplished all that I can and that my work here is now finished. There is nothing else I want to do. I feel that I am just existing as a shell. The person inside has died. The lights have gone out and the person has been mushed to a pulp like a squashed dead insect.

I am looking at me and I seem dead. My hair is straggled and my skin mutilated. My fingers lie solid over the keyboard tapping at random, then resting again in contemplation.

What do I want? I want the winter in my head to thaw. I want the ice to break and for the buds of new thoughts to grow. I want the sunshine back in my heart and the spring in my step. Oh sad thoughts please leave me. I want you out. Out. Out.

I am wrapping my arms around my inner child. I want to come back. Eventually, I will. Like time, this state will pass me by.

Isobel Knight

Discomfort

I am trying not to jump.
The wall is stone and secure against the roar of the
ocean below.
Waves rumble along rhythmically and briskly
They are too busy for emotions.

I am digging the pit of my nail into the flesh of my
arm.
In a restaurant, feeling disgusting, just begging
myself to go,
To be meshed into a pulp by the cauldron beyond,
Willing the ocean to swallow me and my discomfort
whole.

SKIN COLLECTION

Inertia

Musical notes fall upon me. Cold snowflakes.
They touch me as light as feathers and become my
whole world.
I am lying flat upon a cathedral floor, and the space
elevates me.
My eyes soar like trumpets upon fan vaulting and
the roof of Heaven.

The frozen floor restrains me, cold as iron.
Paralysed, I remain as still as death.
I am unbelievably overwhelmed by a power that is
sheer size.
My thoughts tie handcuffs around my wrists and
ankles.

Inside me are bursting grey rain clouds.
Time passes me by, minute by tiny minute.
It is as if I am waiting for something.
To happen.
Cold lingers like a blanket. Death whispers her chill.
Shhh.

There is crimson flowing out of the cathedral floor.
It spews out of the door as if out of a giant mouth.
Outside rain dashes the windows and I cry my first
tears.
As I gaze upward, the world spins on its axis.

Patterns whirl into one another in kaleidoscopic
style.
One colour stands out. Bright. White.

Isobel Knight

Sound waves propel me upwards and my spirit takes flight

SKIN COLLECTION

Mouse Play

"I want to die" said Harvest Mouse.

Seeing that she was serious, the Dormouse cocked her eye at him.

"Are you sure, little thing?"

"I've done all that I want to do and I'm ready to go now."

"What about having children, visiting Fyfield, Farmer Joe's wheat field..."

"I am serious. Lots of mice have children and visiting Fyfield is just a pipe-dream. All I want is Golden Field now."

"But you aren't very old, Harry. You've got several good years in you yet!"

"That is just it – I feel that I have done everything I want to and now it is time."

"Umm. Well some do more in a short life-time than others can do in a vast one. What about your family and friends?"

"I plan to just slip away quietly and not tell them"

"Well that doesn't sound very thoughtful of you – that is a terrible thing to do"

"Oh Dora, please. You make it sound like I am about to commit a crime"

"Well, aren't you?"

"I just can't go on feeling as I do – crushed and angry. Bitter. Desperately sad. I am exhausted of the continuous struggle of life."

"Umm. That is not easy. I can see how troubled you are."

"Harry, I can see you have thought this through but if you were to take your own life, you can't change your mind unless you get help very quickly. What about me – I'll miss you".

"Dora, please – don't get in my way, but understand that although I will be leaving people behind that I love and care about, it is the only way forwards and I don't harbour any regrets".

"Have you thought about how you are going to do it?"

"My death, you mean? Yes, I've thought about it. I really just want to slip away permanently. I just need to find the right berries to take".

"Have you written any notes or letters?"

"Yes, my Will needs a final edit – not that I have much to leave anyone at all. That is just it – I have nothing to show for my life".

"People are more important than material possessions or money. You of all people should know that, Harry. What about your writing?"

"Writing – ha ha. You'll find it all on my laptop. Not the sort of stuff many people would want to read anyway, I should imagine"

"So that is it then. One life-time blown out in a puff of smoke. When are you going to do it then?"

"When am I going to die? When I find the right berries to take. I am going to look upwards and journey towards the Golden Field"

"Are you sure you'd rather not go to Fyfield – I'll pay for your ticket"

"That is kind of you, but my mind is made up and nothing will change my mind. I know that this is a big ask, but will you tell friends and family afterwards that there was nothing that they could have done to dissuade me"

"That is a big thing to ask me. They will want to know why I didn't involve the help of any professionals"

"Dora, the ones who know the most about me know the professionals were involved anyway"

"Harry, I really can't be any further involved, but if the inevitable happens, I will try and explain that your mind was set on this one-way journey. You do know that you can't change your mind once you take the berries?"

"I am fully in control of this particular decision, which is why it feels so right"

"I had noticed that you are no longer interested in new things and the future. You know I will miss you very much, Harry. You are a very special and much-loved mouse"

"I love you too Dora, but this is a journey that I have to see and do alone. I will thing of you on your onward quest to Fyfield. May this year's harvest flourish".

"I won't say goodbye, Harry, but safe onward journey where ever it takes you. I hope that you find peace along the way."

Isobel Knight

Before I go

I wondered what anyone would miss *if* I was gone?
The library would write requesting their books back,
Doctors would be tutting over another DNA,
The cat would be peeved, but it would befriend another human.
Banks would continue to generate reams of trees saying what I owned and owed,
My mobile phone provider would continue to sell me an upgrade,
Parry would be victorious because he no longer had to pay me,
Volunteers would continue to be replaced at work,
Patients would find other therapists to sort out their ills,
My landlady would miss the rent.

I wondered what anyone would miss when *I* was gone?
I would be a name scrubbed out in an address book,
Gmail would reclaim my email address and I would fade from cyberspace.
Some people would ask, did I really go? They hadn't seen me in ages.
Family would miss me, but not forever, I would be a burden relieved.
Friends who were too busy for me in the present, would temporarily grieve my absence, but then I would be out of the loop.
Nothing would change.

I wondered what *I* would miss when I am gone?

SKIN COLLECTION

I would miss the brightness of the sunlight, the flowers and the trees,
Furry animals, especially the warmth of my cat,
The smell of sunshine, sandy beaches, and watching lighthouses at night;
Drinking coffee, eating shortbread and the magic of the moon.
I would miss the deliciousness of hearing music, of laughter and being asleep.

I wondered what I would *not* miss when I am gone?
Feeling hopeless, excruitiatingly sad, exhausted and in pain.
Fighting a never-ending battle against myself.
Fitting in with the world, but never quite managing it,
People bullying me, making me frightened, sad and lonely.
The fact that the good days are over, that our planet is being destroyed.
Negativity, doom and gloom. People's unkindness and poison,
The fact that nothing good ever happens, or lasts for so little time,
Fighting against a tide of negative energy in my life environment.

I wondered what I would like to say *after* I have gone?
It had to be this way. It wasn't you, it was me.
Look after the animals; the birds and the bees
Care for the rivers, the trees and the beauty of the earth

Isobel Knight

Look out for and listen to each other. Where do you
want to go?
I will always be amongst the twinkliest of stars,
always smiling at you.

SKIN COLLECTION

Endings

The final act closed and the swish of the curtains;
Wind blowing the silence at their edges, whispering
about a life God blew out.
Fingers burnt from the extinguished candle.

All around me are walls with nowhere to go; a
dead-end maze.
Out of my hourglass wisp the last few grains of a
life;
I inhale and exhale one last time;
Everything grinds to a halt and I bow out.

Isobel Knight

What Happens at the End?

The end. Two short little words.
Terminal, Finito. Kaput.
Something that is over completely, that will never
again be.
Closed and passed
Finished

SKIN COLLECTION

What am I Doing Here?

An overwhelming heaviness rests in my head, but still pulses of electricity flow through my fingers.
Guilt pulsates in my belly as I wonder what I am here for.

I am full of empty inside and my heart is breaking with the sombre chords of Marcello.
I am at loggerheads with every possible thought, feeling and course of action.

If I were travelling north, I'd want to be south. If I were dancing, I'd prefer to read a book. To be with people, or not. That is the question.
No side of the fence is the 'right' side.

Staring out of the window, I ponder how it all came to be; how things evolved to this point.
I often wonder why things don't grind to a halt. If they did, would life re-start in the same way? Would I arrive for work at 9am?
What makes us keep going? Who are we doing it for?

I can't just live my life getting on with it everyday because I need to understand what it is all about.
Some people say I should just stop worrying about my feelings and thoughts and just 'live'; but there has to be a bigger purpose.

Life is a journey in our bodies, the end of which sees them discarded.
And then what?

Isobel Knight

Some people are obsessed with buying houses and possessions, but I am completely disinterested in this because I can't take these things with me.
The memory bank in my head, and the things I have experienced are more important to me.

People with mental health problems are not crazy, they just see things a bit differently. I feel in constant disharmony with myself because I am battling with why I am alive and what I *should* be doing. I am fracturing more and more relationships because the way other people behave makes me feel more and more uncomfortable.

I don't want to go to parties and celebrations because I find them false, and can't understand why people enjoy them. I don't want to wear special clothes or dress up. I'd like people to see who I am, however exposing that is for them or me.

Sometimes I have forgotten why I like any people at all. They get in my way and interrupt my peace. They are complicated and demanding when I just want simplicity. They overcrowd my head and freak me out.
I behave badly because I'll say the wrong things and sometimes just to be bloody-minded because I am so irritated.

Just sometimes I want to shout really loudly, NO NO NO NO.
Nobody quite sees it my way. I have often wondered how we all see and perceive colours and

sounds; whether square pegs can fit into round holes.

Maybe like the ant that is crawling across my table, I am just making my way though, I can't just be like everybody else, and perhaps that is what bothers me the most. The trouble is that I am now going in such a different direction that I am reaching a point of no return.

I think that one day soon I am going to keep on walking (and writing) but it might be alone, far from the madding crowds. It is not that I won't care for family and friends, it is just that I want to detach myself from the motorway of life. I will just pass through and leave my mark.

Isobel Knight

End O Me Tree O sis

Climb up my tree, Oh Sister.
End
Endometriosis.
Strange word
A Trio of what.

Please end, because if you do not I will. Stop playing trios with my sister.

My tears are free-flowing. You have spoilt things. When I am I going to meet my end with you.

I am curled up in a ball under a tree. The walnuts that are my ovaries are burning like fire and their roots are pulling me into the ground and twisting and turning into many knots.

My face is contorted like the agony of an old tree trunk. An arrow pierces my spine and flays my arms. I wither underground, decaying like the autumn.

The weather is dark grey and still. Every now and then the sky weeps with me. I become concave and the dust of the soil whips over me.

A blackness overtakes me and I am enveloped in codeine. A child above me swings on the bough of a tree. Her lurching jump rebounds upon me.

Cracks in the soil are flooded with my tears. Pain leaks across the fields, but still my innards burn like

SKIN COLLECTION

the embers of an old fire. I am raw. My nerves are like an old fire grate and remember the heat.

Blood flows from me like a young stream. Its energy freaks me as it penetrates every possible tissue source. Its anger radiates like the lava of a volcano.

A man bends down to envelope me in his arms. I cry out that I cannot generate a new-being. My pollen is dead and there will be no new sapling from me.

Above me a surgeon paints my abdomen yellow. Everything goes quiet. The anaesthetic generates white wings of angels.

The deepest cut is made that releases me. Out of it, I am singing. My womb is thrown out like a canon ball and my ovaries bounce like ping-pong balls. The sound makes me laugh.

I am scooped out and hollowed. Where the stitches are new life generates. I come to. My surgeon is smiling. Although I am sore I get up. I am weary, but I have found a new strength.

I am bought a cup of tea. Peace descends over me. I survived. The white wings of a swan beat over me. My soul is full of golden energy.

I get up and walk. I am free.
I am with my sister. I am in a trio.
The O has Ended.

Isobel Knight

The Noise!

The noise. The noise!
Imagine the neighbourhood dog never shuts up,
The perpetual cry of a hungry baby.
Continuous road-digging or a wailing car alarm.
This is the terrible sound of chronic pain.
It is often so loud that I can hardly hear a normal
human conversation.

To match the pain that I am experiencing I might
down six vodka and tonics,
Burn myself with an iron, rip my skin, down some
morphine, or destroy a room.
There is a roaring fire inside me that wants me to
grind the hot coals of pain to powder.
If I could scream loud enough, the road outside
would rip apart.
The guts of the earth would embowel and be
strewn over the street.

A drill bores into my lower back.
The pain here is so intensely focussed I could nail
it.
The pain in my pelvis is blunt. Broad. Flat. Dull.
Laboured. Heavy. Grey.
Two areas each the size of stones feel sore and
tender. They resonate.
The pain in my middle pulls me down like the
weight of a rock.
Like an injured animal I crawl, dragging all this with
me everywhere I go.

SKIN COLLECTION

Pain - Embers

For just a moment on waking, it is perfect. I am peaceful and calm.
And then I remember.

The gnawing pain in my pelvis jolts me, nerves cranking into action and another day begins.

I groan with fatigue as my mind flips through a mental checklist of the day ahead, whilst managing my body.

It would be so much easier to battle with my duvet than to drag my unwilling body throughout the day.

Attached to my hands and feet are a ball and chain. The embers in my pelvis are stoked up for the day and we are full-steam ahead.

I shove a few pills in my mouth and a heat-pad on my belly and prepare for an endurance test.

In my head the tortoise plods along with grim determination.

I too wait to retreat in my shell, dying to curl up in a ball.

As the lights fade out, I am peaceful and calm.
And then I forget.

Isobel Knight

"To You"

I look at you and know that you are hurting; I can see the pain in your eyes and the drops forming at the corner of your eyes ooze vulnerability. I gather you up in my arms like a bundle of wood, being careful not to splinter you. We are sitting in bed and I am behind you with my legs around yours in the 'spoon embrace'. I am kissing you tenderly, but non-sexually on the nape of the neck, and stroking your hair. I am rocking you rhythmically, but oh, so gently. The bravery in your face is being washed away by your flowing tears. I want you to let it all out. I stroke your arms and my silence intensifies as I listen to your broken words. Gradually I am anchoring you, and although you are still a heaving wreck, you have let go and let me take you on board.

Gradually you subside, and your storm tempers. I gently cover us both with a quilt and you crash in my arms; exhausted by your fight. Your breathing relaxes like a subtle breeze, and I cease rocking you. I place you gently onto your side and wrap my being around yours, until we are a jigsaw, saving any missing pieces. I continue to stroke your soft, warm body, before I myself succumb to sleep.

SKIN COLLECTION

Bile

My fist clamps tightly shut in the form of a clam.
My finger-tips are a rubber seal and the blood
drains out grey.
My flesh is frigid cold.

Sweat leaks like pus and oozes like an abscess.
I'm putrid with anger.
My teeth are set-wide and saliva drips slowly like a
stalagmite.
My mouth tastes as bitter as gall.

Energy pounds me in the stomach, and I throw a
cannon
The stretch violates my calves and I slide down a
hill.
The epidermis leaves my finger-tips.
I kick into next Christmas.

Ricocheting and turning, I cascade downward
bound.
Up-thrown by potholes and moles.
Momentum and energy gather,
I pause, lying upward and laugh.

Serious now, for he has a foot on my stomach,
I sober and solidify like a statue.
Weight crushes my innards and they reek out of my
mouth.
The black hole left inside screams.
Silence.

Clods of earth cover me like moss.

Isobel Knight

My voice, useless in life, vomits in the darkness.
My hysteria is heard.
I scratch the eyes out of the clouds.

SKIN COLLECTION

Snake Dance

Inside things spiralled.
A spherical body coiled round and round itself,
becoming increasingly taut.
The maraca on her tail clearly agitated.
Eyes were fixated, poised and bore like gimlets.
Venom seething and finally she struck her prey with
virulent fury

The victim was clearly stunned as the life drained
out of his eyes,
She slid away, still in a temper, flashing fire, with
beasts clearing her track
Hacking venom from the devil's pit, poison squirted
recklessly.
Gradually her dance subsided and gracefully she
slipped away.
Things spiralled outside.

Isobel Knight

The Worry Organ

It is located in the fleshy part, below the sternum.
The size of my heart, with the flatness of my hand.
Dark, purple and constant,
Fluttering with the eloquence of a toad.

Pressure tightens across my worry organ,
It is as subtle as a blunt vegetable knife.
All consuming, it sucks the calm out of me,
A nest of anxieties keeps me buzzing.

SKIN COLLECTION

Waiting

I sat and waited for you by the window.
I wasn't seeing, I bit away the crescent of my thumb,
My knuckles merely grazed my cheek bones, elbows collapsed upon my knees.
I felt utterly grounded; my legs creating a bridge from my buttocks.

A drip of moisture made soggy my knuckles,
I flicked the juice out of my eyes, the back of my hand an inadequate tissue.
My thumb remained on edge lest I should attack it again.
My eyes were blurred with clarity.

At gut level, I was struck hemispherically.
It cut me with a cheese wire – that I couldn't see him.
His fist gouged my diaphragm,
The squeeze was unbearable.

The hump in my back echoes the droop of my lips
My ears fantasise the return of his steps, my nerves; the sense of his touch.
A whole drama is unfolding outside the window;
Of the night he died in the soaking wet rain.

Isobel Knight

Separation

My inner core has been scooped out,
A void so large has been left,
Tears split me in two.

My heart is bled out,
A dagger has skewered me right,
The pain is so great.

SKIN COLLECTION

Regret

Regret poured out of her mouth,
In rhythmical, even spurts

Sorry, sad, symmetrical, solitary
Stupid, small sounds

She asked for forgiveness, although the die was cast.
No one was waive ring her behaviour.

To erase time would be too much to ask,
Un-walking a virginal journey.

Just not-knowing would be enough,
It was too late for if only.

She had dug her own grave, and was being buried by the shovelful,
Lying, choking on her own error, she felt compelled to

Spew; irony and appalling disbelief.
She had initiated her death.

Treatment stopped by one who had cared,
betrayed by avenged action.
What you did was wrong, wrong, wrong.

She was the loser now and when rank took hold,
She was left out in the cold.

Exposed, shamed and named

Isobel Knight

The door in her face, rammed.

(All) she did was to say what she felt and held to be real.
It would have been (far) better for her lips to seal.

SKIN COLLECTION

Once Bitten

I don't know when I realised it.
Just as a sly fox upon the hen, it crept up slowly.

When the jaws bit in, their indentions left,
Scorching marks and floods of desire.

That person on a sun-bed lay,
Their profile etched as my footprint upon the sand.

I stared up the white walls as my memory recalled,
A catalogue of information about them.

I am now in a feverish anxiety, waiting for them.
My pulse is in a bloody hurry.

O quickly come!
Lock me in your embrace.

Isobel Knight

Oh Love

Oh Love,
You rip and tug at my chest wall, like Velcro.
Like a plaster, I pull you off bit by bit, letting blood
seep between my fingers,
Flowing like a river, draining me of energy, you
gather like a well at my feet.

My thoughts flutter like a butterfly and tension
lingers in my belly.
I want to kiss you.

SKIN COLLECTION

Leonora (Fictional name)

Oh Leonora, darling.
You have put me under a
Spell with your deep brown eyes,
Honest face and wide-open smile. I
Love your warmth, your caring and concern.
I remember you put your arm around me once. I
Wanted you to envelop me with your whole live
body.
You listen and it is real. You care and it is genuine.
You act
With interest and give me your fullest attention. You
focus on the now.

You interact with humour, wit and intelligence. You
exude great empathy.
It was good to see you today. You looked older,
wiser and thoughtful.
I have never forgotten all that you have done for me
over the years.
There seems to be an invisible pull between us. A
silent and
Energetic force. Words maybe left unsaid, but
silence and
Gesture show there is something there. I feel you
like
Me. And want to get to know more about me too.
I love your intellectual look and approach.
I want to kiss and embrace you.
Do you feel the same?
Oh Leonora, darling.

Isobel Knight

Impatience – or why I am one fucked-up Love Bunny

Someone tore at the curtains of my heart.
My hand is stretched out fully to crisis, I never made contact with them.

Misery grazes my face, a rope is uncoiled from the pit of my stomach, unravelling down the road.

Screams pierce the darkness in my head and whistle out of my skull.

I want him, oh god.

Like a sacrifice I am lain dead at her feet.
I would dance naked down the street, turn Catherine wheels until the flames sparkle the skies and ignite us.

Jumping Jack in somersault, reach and pull me down,
Over and over, I flip, upside down. A flat gingerbread, who has been caught by the wolf.

In flight I soar the foggy skies that cloud my comprehension.

I turn inside out, agony unscrews in the darkness.
Wax is dripping out of my formless self.

The clock moves so reluctantly I have to budge it with the second hand.

SKIN COLLECTION

MOVE.

I want closer lands. She is a billion miles away from me.
In a mirror dance I am dressing in the body suit that unites us.

As I zip up, the cords bind my heart-strings and heal me in my bloody wait for her.

I just sit at the window, allowing my gazing eyes to immerse into the mist.

Isobel Knight

Old Lover

In her hands she tightly ground fine sand,
Grains released in a vortex, wisps of her life,
each a significant memory.

Lightly wavy, the breeze blew her hair, softly, softly.
Sunshine smarted her cheeks, blue eyes glistening
with dew;
The sea foam a fresh ejaculation.
Waves moan and shudder in release, like an old
lover

SKIN COLLECTION

Tonsil Hockey

Tongues whirling like a washing machine
Spinning faces

Lashing

Slurping and suction
Dribbling juices in the rinse cycle

Free-flowing

Rubbery lips folding over each other
In the mix of the wash

Teeth hit
And miss

Foaming at the mouth
Lover's suds throth

And love goes around and around

Isobel Knight

In a (Inner) lather

It was feverish and hot in there,
We were revolving like rolling pins;
Our hands ravenous for touch
A duo of grace overturned.

Urgency enveloped the room,
Limbs entwined each other, pulling at their roots.
Breath was rapid and gasping,
The release was ultimate and timely.

SKIN COLLECTION

Love is….

Sticky toffee pudding and ice-cream
A glorious rainbow
The mew of a kitten
Striations from a harp
Fresh coffee

Delightful
Hilarious
Sublime
Idyllic

Rolling down a hill
Uncontrollable laughter
Infectious energy
Hot and evolving
Continuous

Isobel Knight

Breaking Point

I should have known it was going to happen
The day before I felt the warning signals;
A siren beeping in my leg
Just a minute!

In one space I am dancing fantastically,
My body is responding beautifully to all the instructions
Fluent, free-flowing and seamless sequences
My whole form extended in curvaceous lines.
Then.

It just snapped. I heard the tear.
The end grounded me, and I swept my body from the floor.
Pain seared in my calf, and I just wanting to howl.
All I could see was the wall and weeks of no ballet.

It is the end of the world, and is so unfair.
People crowd around who care, but they are really thinking, "thank God it wasn't me"
My life changed in one second.
The point that broke my leg.

SKIN COLLECTION

Still no Allegro

My feet absorb the ground,
Sponge-like;
Toes are webbing,
Arches support.

I go through my feet to a point,
They are a smiling-crescent;
Together they rise on to demi-pointe,
I am levitated.

Both feet propel me into orbit,
Individually, they may not.
Too weak to go solo;
I may not hop, skip or dart.

Still no allegro.

Isobel Knight

Recital

In the end she didn't need kicking at all.
She walked with great poise and took her place.
There were no rabbit-dazzling lights
Isobel wasn't trapped.

With composure she faced the enemy.
A sideways look at her accompanist; she took an in-breath.
Energetic melodic activity exhaled,
Her fingers a-jigging to a galliard.

The next notes were an Air in G.
Sombre, sedate striations of notes,
Anxious to fulfil their length
Echoed around the church.

The recorder played like a legend.
She savoured rests sweetly.

SKIN COLLECTION

Texture

Nurtured of muslin, cradled that soft, palpable head,
Satin laced tiny fingers in your cot;
Corduroy trousers were patched up at the knees from your tumbles;
Woolly bobble hat knocked off its perch from a flying snowball.

The uniformity of cotton disciplined you,
Leather shoes you wore, with pink ones for ballet;
A red cardigan scratched your delicate skin,
Slipperiness was the silk of your blue bridesmaid dress.

You learnt to crochet, sew and darn;
Embroidery wove its way knitting your life together.
A myriad of colours threaded through your journey;
You have taken the rough with the smooth.

Your warm ivory skin exudes delicacy,
The coarseness and the chaos of your hair exudes energy;
You interlock fingers of lace with your lover,
Contrasting textures bind you together;
The Tapestry of your life unravels…..

Isobel Knight

Up and Down

Public transport grinds,
Covered by a tired old system;
They only have a stained carpet.

Other countries blocked together
Cope with deep steps and heavy snowfalls
That manage to lead to my room.

Here in handrail,things are rickety.
The UK has a few banisters missing
White stuff causes an evenly spaced transport
meltdown.

Given and worn and underneath,
We had been warned the carpet is a wooden floor
of snow
The stairwell is lit above the rate of inflation

Appalling levels of service exist on the first floor
It is quite beyond the average level of stairs,
That we can justify the gradient
Continuing to remove furniture up and down.
I tread carefully.

SKIN COLLECTION

White

Spiky and short,
One syllable long,
You come with light against a silhouette.

Blatant and evil,
Two serenading doves,
You hit between W and E.

Ghostly and pointed,
Three blind mice,
You completely daunt me.

Isobel Knight

Moon

Magical and magnificent;
Round and embracing femininity;
She radiates silvery grey;
A light of varying intensity

She points the way, a stage-light for life.
Her shape changing cyclically,
Choosing to expose herself as a gigantic circle, or
crescent;
Mystery surrounds her;
She wears a cloak of stars.

The night is eerie;
Silence is suspending the darkness,
Your beam dispels fear and oozes serenity
You were once in my dreams.

SKIN COLLECTION

Haiku of The Moon

A light of varying intensity
She points the way, a stage-light for life.
You were once in my dreams.

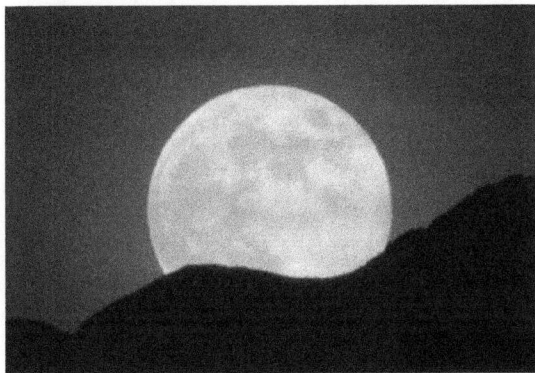

Isobel Knight

Kali

It has almost been a week
Since I stroked your soft black fur,
Burrowed my face in the warm-bread scent of your tummy,
Let you lick my paw.

It has almost been a week since you
Howled at me because you had got lost
Chirruped at me when you felt my embrace
Purred when I stroked your g-spot

Time will not fade the glossiness of your coat,
The memory of your army of whiskers,
Or those beautiful, but blind golden eyes.
Nor your sweet nature, or dainty and gentle approach.

We didn't know each other long, but we *had* each other.
Your calm and inner wisdom, for my bed and Go-Cat
Every day I still look for you,
Your presence will always be.

SKIN COLLECTION

Horatio

An army thud signifies your arrival,
Your eyes, pleading with mine,
A whimper of miaow passes your whiskery chops,
as delicate as the blow of a feather,
Diamonds on your tail march onto the waves of
your back.

You sit, and are not backing down.
The arcs of your mouth are firmly down and you will
not be moved.
Stoutly you defend your sofa.
Lethal hooks in your claws swipe your territory.

When you jump, the earth moves. Elegance is not
your grace.
Built to scare, yet in need of a cuddle yourself,
Your ear touches my cheek with tenderness,
The vibration of your purr, a 6.8 on the Richter
scale.

Solidly you mould my lap.
You have owned it all your life.
Tufts of your fur lovingly float around.
Your Majesty owns this place.

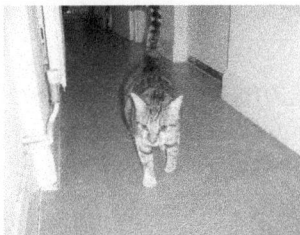

Isobel Knight

My Birthday

Once upon a time, there had been plenty of space.
It was warm and safe in there, and slowly you grew.
And grew.

Your due date came and went, and you had to
become a contortionist.
You were bound tightly into a ball, and oxygen
became a luxury.

A tidal wave crushed you in half and took the wind
out of your lungs,
You were in agony, and wondered what you had
done to deserve this.

Terror struck, and enveloped you in panic.
There had to be a way out of this menacing space.

You went through hours of crashing waves,
battering your tiny body,

Until

You saw the way.

Your body twisted and turned, and you were
petrified all the time.

In the distance was a half-crescent of orange light
and you kicked with all your might, and emerged.

In one move you were born, and celebrated by
inhaling the breath of your life.

SKIN COLLECTION

First Thing

S-T-R-E-T-C-H!
I pull the sleep out of my arms,
My eyes fling open
My feet wait to dance away the day

A light-bulb of anticipation flickers in my belly
Happiness swamps my face
Excitement electrifies me
It is the weekend!

Isobel Knight

In Extension

Flying up to catch my heart,
My arms gesture towards the sun,
My happiness is completely unreachable,
Rainbow smiles fill my face.

The first time I point my foot,
A stretch arches throughout my being from tip to
toe;
Poise pulls up through my head,
Puppet strings coordinate my movements.

As I am bent in half, my hamstrings sing;
Joy seeps through my pores; beads of sweat
dance.
I am moved from pose to pose.
Flying melodies transport my delight.

In a spin now, I am beautifully disconnected;
Elegance in soaring leaps, and the beauty of
arabesque;
I am in the flow of movement,
Transformed by the magic of dance.

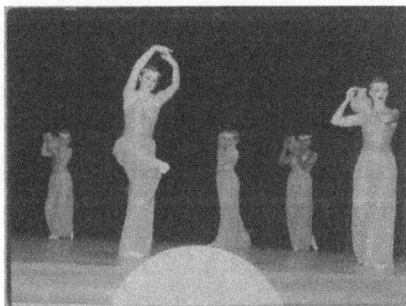

SKIN COLLECTION

My classical ballet teacher

A swan elegance of theatrical black, punctuated
with silver,
The epitome of style.

Her hair, a silky black in a chiselled bob;
Angular and quizzical, her expression;
Poise radiates from her smile.

Beautifully connected, her body makes all the right
moves;
She has the grace and dynamics of a panther,
Her movements are sleek with precision.

A wonderful inspiration; she deserves the greatest
respect.

Isobel Knight

Ecstatic

Happiness radiated.
It suspended her in thin air
Her smile touched you deep inside
As penetrating as treacle
I licked sugar off my lips

SKIN COLLECTION

Ha Ha

It started in ripples
Bubbling like an excited brook
Quaking her sides,
Rocking to and fro,
It was *so* funny

Isobel Knight

High

A rainbow smile she wore,
A coat of many colours.
Her happiness was contagious
Joy danced all around

SKIN COLLECTION

Review of CAT Therapy

I am 34 years old. This in itself is of minor insignificance until it is substantiated by the fact I have been self-harming for 27 of those 34 years.

Nobody, least of all me knows precisely when I started to self-harm in the form of skin-picking. I know that I was about 5 years old and had already started to take immense dislike to my skin, which was weepy and flaky in parts (mainly joints) related to excema. After this I started to pick other skin abrasions or spots, such as mosquito bites. These spots increased in size, from tiny dots to much larger marks, and every time the skin healed these spots, I would pick the scab off them continually until the area of skin eventually scarred.

Until I was about 8 or 9 years old, these 'spots' would occur on my lower and upper limbs only, and there would be possibly up to three or four 'sites' at a time. From thereon in, spots started to appear on my face and again the number could be up to two or three of these sites and by the time I was 12, the size of these sites had sometimes increased dramatically – there were incidents of spots as large as the old fifty pence pieces.

By the time I was 15 I had all but stopped picking my face, but nevertheless continued to self-harm picking my head and scalp instead often having sizeable areas of baldness and scabby skin. The picking elsewhere on the body diminished, although picking on the lower limbs did not stop until I was part the way through my CAT therapy.

When I was growing up, there was no mention of the words self-harm as we now know and understand them. Instead, my skin-picking was referred to as a habit, or a 'Compulsive Behavioural Disorder'. Whilst the skin-picking did undoubtedly relieve feelings of anxiety and upset, it was still not mentioned as an act of self-harm.

At 12 years old I was sent to a child psychologist (Dr S) who I (now) believe used a CBT (Cognitive Behavioural Therapy) approach to her sessions. At the time I used to rebel against the sessions and deliberately lied in the diary I was supposed to use to record the feelings before and after I picked. Neither did I find relaxation techniques particularly helpful. Dr S often wrongly attributed my skin-picking to my father's death. My father had died five years after this behaviour had started.

It has been my experience that the medical profession can get things wrong nearly as often as they get them right. Even when they are right, it can still be a battle-ground to sort things out. I am therefore quite angry that it has taken until very recently to explain that my skin-picking is a form of self-harm and more importantly, to look at how or why I have been doing this, and how I can in fact stop this behaviour.

In writing this article, I have no reason to portion blame or otherwise to my family, in particular my mother and my younger sister who watched me single-handedly destroy my skin. My mother, often very angry *at* me, was obviously hurting about the actions I was taking over myself, rather than angry *with* me as a person. I can now see this crucial difference.

Either way, it seems that at one point or another in my development, I found skin-picking as a way in which to cope with difficult and painful thoughts and emotions; In other words, taking direct action over myself helped me to relieve some of the discomfort of certain strong feelings and emotions – such as anger, sadness and anxiety.

For me there was also the added adrenaline factor in that I would also be punished for having picked. This would increase my anxiety and thus increase the amount of picking I did.

Over the years I was able to completely detach my body from my head and mind to the extent that I no longer felt any pain from the course of my actions. This also meant that I could find increasing other ways to hurt myself such as hitting myself, head-banging and later on taking an overdose.

External to the skin-picking were increased mood-swings, depression, increased feelings of unresolved anger and difficulties in handling relationships of any kind.

There were several occasions throughout my life when I was in need of 'talking therapies'. Indeed I had a year of psychotherapy from 2001-2, but this was unable to address the self-harm in any way or form. Neither did the tools of CBT which were learnt on a pain management programme as well as a one-to-one session with a therapist.

When I started CAT (Cognitive Analytical Therapy), I was initially positive about it, although because I felt generally well at the time, I thought it would be another talking therapy and perhaps another unproductive waste of time.

One of the first things I did with Dr H (my CAT Therapist) was to identify the different moods that I could get into that caused me to feel uncomfortable and then ultimately self-harm. When I became quite good at this, we looked at how I could get into different states with people – perhaps feeling controlled, or angry, and then I would turn to self-harm as a way of dealing with this feeling rather than discussing it directly with the other person.

In addition to that, it was also noted that I could go into a completely numb and detached state which was when the self-harm often took place. One of the most important aspects of the therapy was to involve me getting back in touch with my real physical body and all it's sensations; the good and the bad. This was particularly hard for me given that I suffer from a chronic and sometimes very painful condition called 'Endometriosis'.

Dr H and I also realised that I could get into some other difficult states with people which could mean that I either idolised or loathed them. This was often the case where my own care needs were not being met, or if I had particularly strong feelings of love towards a person, which was often unrequited, or fantastical. I also learned that I could be quite manipulative towards other people which was another unpleasant revelation.

One of the biggest learning curves involved looking at the way in which I communicated with people. For instance telling them I am angry, or unhappy or sad and why; rather than leaving them to guess, or worse, be left with no opportunity to tell them at all. We agreed that this action had to be addressed verbally rather than in my preferred form of written communication.

We did decide that writing was a very important way in which I could put down in words difficult feelings that I did not yet want to talk about and would give me the necessary distance from the self-harm.

Once I began to understand the link between the unpleasant feelings and the self-harm, and also to get back 'into' my body, it has finally meant that my self-harm has radically reduced and I have already had days and weeks when I have not self-harmed at all. Given that it is still early days, I am still very encouraged with the results and the tools that I learned in CAT therapy.

I am quite proud of myself that I have sometimes coped with the same bad feelings I have always had – e.g. anger, but not self-harmed and done something else instead, perhaps writing or dancing. There have been slip-ups, but I am into the first few years of changing a 27 year old method of coping with thoughts and emotions. Strangely enough, I have also felt occasional loss in my habit, but looking much better and being proud of my body is definitely winning. I am also feeling better in myself, gradually at last becoming comfortable in my own skin.

One of the biggest problems that still remains is that I can suffer from quite significant mood swings and although I am not necessarily self-harming to escape them, I am finding them very hard to cope with; particularly an overwhelming depression that sometimes strikes.

I am about to have my medication changed, coming of an SSRI, Duloxetine and changing to a mood-stablising drug, Lamotrigine. There is no doubt that even if this helps, the tools of CAT will still be very important, coupled with an increasingly sophisticated way of coping with difficult feelings and improved ways of relating to other people.

"Getting back in Touch"

Before it was just two separate circles. There was my body, and there was my mind, and they were two completely different entities. It seemed that my head was severed from my body, and my body felt no pain that I inflicted upon it.

However deeply I dug my fingers and pulled at the healing wound of skin, my body was completely numb and only the leaking crimson could possibly alert me to any danger. There was always that moment of tension when my fingers prised off the edge of that crust; that sparkle underneath, glistening like a trophy. The relief when it was over was like that latest cigarette, and my craving was satisfied. Minutes later, there would be pain, but again, I would sever this in my head and carry my wound with me.

The first thing that practically helped me to stop self-injuring myself was to start by befriending my skin. To start with, I found it hard to actually look at it; live it and experience it's texture, it's warmth, it's living. It took a long time to feel comfortable touching my skin, not wanting to hack at it.

I started to use moisturising cream. First on my shins which were in the worst mess at the time. It started by buying some E45 Lotion, and after every bath or shower, I would apply three pump ejections of this 500ml of Lotion to each leg from the knee below. To start with I still couldn't bear to touch this part of my leg. I just flung on the cream, but with no real love or care. It took effort to do this and even though I knew from my Life Coaching work that it would take at least 21 days for this habit to become ingrained, I didn't enjoy it initially.

Once this daily act became habit, I started to be able to look at the results and the quality of the skin on my shins. I still had some picking sites on them, but the other skin was starting to feel silkier, and instead of just rushing to apply the cream, I started to pay more attention to how it actually felt; and so I started to put some actual love into the creaming act.

Gradually there were less 'sites' on my legs and eventually I realised that I was finally picking a bit less. It took me a long time to appreciate that this was because I was starting to experience a sensation of feeling in my skin and that my skin really and truly was a part of me; like it or not.

At this point, I realised that my body and mind were no longer completely separate entities, but they were actually joined, and so my two very separate circles became a Venn Diagram.[1] By this time, I also started to apply moisturiser cream to other parts of my body. I had applied cream to my face for many years as part of a very basic beauty regime, but had never considered that my whole body might appreciate the application of cream.

---

[1] The Venn Diagram is made up of two or more overlapping circles. It is often used in mathematics to show relationships between sets. In language arts instruction, Venn Diagrams are useful for examining similarities and differences in characters, stories, poems, etc.

SKIN COLLECTION

It felt extraordinary after all this time showing my body some care. Again it took me many attempts before I felt remotely comfortable in touching my body in various places. Any places. It made me wonder how I ever coped in doing a physical body therapy such as 'The Bowen Technique', and touching other people's bodies, or in allowing previous lovers to touch my body. It made me realise that if I could really start to feel comfortable in my own skin, it might make me feel more relaxed and start to enjoy my body and start loving it. Gradually I started to feel more real. I won't pretend it was easy, because it took quite a lot of practice to start substituting creating harm on my body for healthier behaviours such as applying love and cream to my body. Once I had got used to applying cream to my body, I started stroking it with no cream on it. This was harder as I felt the real skin under my finger-tips, imperfections and all. This meant that I panicked when I found rough skin and would remove it, but actually in a lot less vicious an attack.

Eventually I was picking less because when I tried to pick my skin, it actually started to cause me pain, and the pain itself would increasingly stop me wanting to rip any scabs from the surface. The fact I could finally feel the pain of my actions was a massive breakthrough, and it was in this revelation that I started to get inside my body, and the two initially very separate circles of mind and body overlapped some more.

Isobel Knight

Slowly my body started to belong to me. My originally 'Lego' head had to be screwed well and truly onto my body suit. I started to use simple actions like stroking the backs of my hands as a way of coping if I felt stressed or anxious because this sensation kept me fixed on my skin and feeling 'real' and keeping in touch and 'in my body' so I could feel that it was a pleasant and pain-free sense of touch. This reinforced a feeling of calm and kept my attacking levels down to the bare minimum.

In the early days there were still many times when the above strategies were unhelpful as that long habit of causing myself pain and inflicting injury was so well entrenched, it was going to take months of practice to undo this automatic action. Even now (nine months later) I still have episodes where I still go into attack mode, and the only times this is really occurring now is when I experience physical pain in my body – such as the pain caused by my endometriosis.

It seems to me that I just cannot handle my body firing off real and genuine pain signals, not ones that I haven't self-induced. It is going to take some time before I truly stop adding an additional level of pain to my body by self-harming it on top of pain signals that it is already sending out in distress. At this point my body really needs as much love as I can afford to give it, and this is where I have started to ask the help of friends.

SKIN COLLECTION

When I am in real physical pain through illness in my own body, I am, as yet, unable to cope with this pain and the anger I feel towards my body is still unfortunately expressed through some degree, albeit minor, of self-harm; usually through a bit of scalp-picking, or hair-pulling. If I am completely unable to relax myself and care for my body just a little, I am finding that if people are able to hold me, hug or cuddle me, I am able to relax a little bit, which also means my true pain-sensations drop a little, and I am less likely to attack and harm myself.

In a way, their sensation of gentle touch subdues me just like the stroking of an anxious furry animal. It is hard because I need at some level to be kept inside my body, even if I want to sever it from my mind, but just enough so that I will not become any more angry with the pain caused through illness, but also because I need to accept and 'feel' that pain.

I believe it will be a while before I can completely sort this last part out, but the rest is extremely encouraging. Before I started therapy I was picking three or four times a day. Minimum. Now I am picking less than three or four times a week, so much so I can forget all about my skin and its imperfections, and instead I am even enjoying its sensations, and am just about tolerating being in it and owning it.

I am hoping that in time the automatic response of attempting to harm my skin will be completely be replaced by the habit of being completely inside it and showing it both unconditional love and respect.

I am well on the way to doing this and have been amazed at how different this feels, and that I could ever be reunited in mind and body. I now quite like wearing my head!

SKIN COLLECTION

Consultation with a Plastic Surgeon

It took me an enormous amount of courage to do it.
To ask my GP to make a referral to see a
Consultant Plastic Surgeon at a time with
increasing cutbacks and tightened purse-strings on
the NHS. My GP, although sympathetic, wasn't
sure whether anyone would see me, but had no
problem in sending me to see someone, and a
referral was subsequently made.

What had been difficult for me in requesting an
appointment was that I was valuable and important
enough a person to be considered worthy of any
such treatment; that any doctor worth his salt would
deem it reasonable to spend time and resources on
a woman who had self-destructed herself. It wasn't
as though I had been involved in a car crash, or
had a burn-related accident.

When I saw the Plastic Surgeon, I was surprised by
how sensitively I was treated. I was asked which
scars on my face that particularly bothered me, and
the doctor had a good look. He then asked me all
about my self-harm; how long it had been going on
for, and where things were at now following the
successful Cognitive Analytical Therapy.

At no point was I made to feel that everything was
my fault and that I was a worthless waste of space.
In fact, just the opposite. I was asked about what I
did work-wise and how I felt about myself. I said
how much more in tune with my body I felt, and

how I was now treating it with a lot more respect and care.

The Plastic Surgeon explained how scar revision would never make the scars go away, but might improve their appearance. Given that my scars were now about 18 years old, he felt that the tissue had blended with my other skin as well as physically possible, but that with the scars on my nose and forehead, a 50% improvement might be possible, but that there wasn't very much chance of improvement to the scars on my cheeks. He also explained how following any surgery that the scars would be quite raised and red for up to six months, and that this might be difficult for me to cope with seeing them red and raw. He then offered me the alternative, which was to see the Red Cross Camouflage Clinic who specialise in treating patients with bad scarring, and have special creams that can be applied to hide scarring. For me this was a very positive suggestion, and I asked him to refer me.

The conclusion of the appointment was that he would consider revising two of my scars if that was what I wanted, if I wasn't happy with the results of the camouflage creams. To me, the latter option this seemed a better solution than the surgery, as certainly the scars looking red and angry again for months was not a great prospect. The consultant also said he would need a report from my therapist to ask her opinion about whether I would be a suitable candidate for any potential surgery. The consultation ended up with me being offered a follow-up appointment for the end of April, if required.

At no point did I really feel during the consultation that I needed to go to confession and say, 'Bless me Father, for I have sinned'. There is a perpetual cycle of apology in self-harmers. They create mess on or to themselves in whatever capacity. They then have to get other people, most often medics to fix their mess – whether it is wrists which require re-stitching, or a stomach to be pumped. It is a destructive cycle and sometimes medics treat self-harmers with great contempt because they know in a cynical way that they will patch up a person only to see them again in A&E a few months later. Some doctors even deny self-harmers pain relief when they stitch them up, saying that if they didn't manage to feel it the first time, they won't now. Fortunately this is now happening much less often.

The secret, as I am learning, is to have worth in yourself, and that you deserve better than to be treating yourself in such a destructive way. Liking yourself is a vital part of this, and once I started to use creams and lotions on myself and start to reconnect with my skin, I started to appreciate that not only could I be an attractive person, potentially, but that I was worth investing time and care on; hence the confidence required to request a Plastic Surgery appointment.

The fact is that I still feel a tremendous sense of guilt about what I did to my skin, but also a sense of sadness. There is a story behind every scar on my face, but beyond that I must hold on to the fact that there really is a lovely and worthwhile person underneath it. I feel very sad now that I messed up my face, and I have to wear my face every day, but instead of hiding behind a mask of mess, I can emphasise my good points such as my eyes and teeth, and to an extent make-up can do the rest. The most important thing now is how I feel about myself on the inside, and that is now doing 90% of the work in facing the world.

SKIN COLLECTION

Postscript

I am sometimes surprised by just how far I have come. It is now 2 years since I finished CAT (Cognitive Analytical Therapy) and the prognosis is now really good. I haven't been harming myself in all that time. This is a remarkable achievement and for me has been an opportunity to re-start my life and put self-harming well and truly behind me. I had been harming for 27 years, so for the first time in my life I feel free. It feels good to be me, and my body and mind finally feel at one.

My thinking, which was so fractured, and black and white; has developed tones of grey and rationality. The way I cope with difficult feelings has improved upon recognition. I am now able to say when I feel anger, or any emotion which previously might have caused me to turn against myself. I relate much better to others as a result. It amused me that on my 34th birthday (December 2008), I had asked a few people from my ballet class if they would like to go out for a drink. I had not told them it was for my birthday. As a result, and because it was such late notice, nobody could come. I wasn't upset. It actually made me smile; it made me realise I am a worthwhile person, and that I still need to improve my communication. This year I will tell everyone at least two weeks beforehand, and advertise it on Facebook!

Right now, I am busy. Very busy. I am finally doing something I am absolutely passionate about. I have my writing, and will always use that as a very positive way of coping against difficult times as they will inevitably present themselves in the future. I am presently studying for an MSc in Dance Science at an incredibly exciting and wonderful space that is Laban. I feel there that I have 'come home'. I therefore very much hope to be able to stay at Laban upon conclusion of my course; working in research, or studying for a PhD. I am so thrilled to be combining so many of my passions; research, writing, classical ballet, and studying the body, in a scientific and medical way. It really doesn't get any better for me. It is a perfect symbiosis of intellectual body and for me in so many other ways. I said earlier that body and mind are one wholly functioning unit.

Finally, I cannot close without reflecting on where I was before without offering hope to the millions of people who have mental health problems. Everyone has different coping strategies, but for me part of that was about believing that I was worthwhile in being helped. It wasn't my fault I self-harmed all those years; I didn't know how to process difficult emotions or feelings in a safe way. I still find it hard to say "I'm feeling low", but I know how to ask for help, or I can recognise that however bad I am feeling on a particular day/week, that the negative feeling will pass, eventually. Countless experience has shown that just like passing clouds, depression (in the form of mood swings) does go away, and then the sun comes out again. My writing is very clear about this.

SKIN COLLECTION

If I can give hope to anybody else who has suffered from mental health problems, then that would be the best possible outcome of this book.

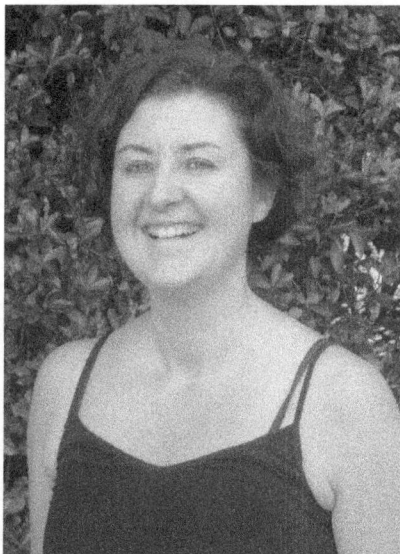

Isobel Knight

www.ingramcontent.com/pod-product-compliance
Lightning Source LLC
Chambersburg PA
CBHW031216270326
41931CB00006B/588